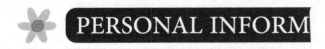 **PERSONAL INFORM**

MW00934835

Name:	
Address:	City:
State/Zip:	Home Phone:
Word Phone:	Cell Phone:

HEIGHT: .... WEIGHT: .... BMI: ....

BLOOD GROUP	

EMERGENCY CONTACTS

Name:	
Address:	City:
State/Zip:	Home Phone:
Word Phone:	Cell Phone:
Relationship:	

Name:	
Address:	City:
State/Zip:	Home Phone:
Word Phone:	Cell Phone:
Relationship:	

Caregiving Notes For: .... **Date:** .... / .... / ....

Toileting							
	Time						
	U						
	BM						

Times up During The Night				

Breakfast	
AM Snack	
Lunch	
PM Snack	
Dinner	
Drinks	

ACTIVITIES & OTHER COMMENTS

Appointments: ....

Health Concerns: ....

Plans For Tommorow: ....

Pain Level: .... Happiness Level: .... Alertness Level: ....

Supplies Needed Soon: ....

Medication Taken: ....

NOTES

Caregiving Notes For: _____ **Date:** _____ / _____ / _____

Toileting	Time							
	U							
	BM							

Times up During The Night				

Breakfast	
AM Snack	
Lunch	
PM Snack	
Dinner	
Drinks	

ACTIVITIES & OTHER COMMENTS

Appointments: _____

Health Concerns: _____

Plans For Tommorow: _____

Pain Level: _____ Happiness Level: _____ Alertness Level: _____

Supplies Needed Soon: _____

Medication Taken: _____

NOTES

Caregiving Notes For: .... **Date:** .... / .... / ....

Toileting	Time							
	U							
	BM							

Times up During The Night				

Breakfast	
AM Snack	
Lunch	
PM Snack	
Dinner	
Drinks	

ACTIVITIES & OTHER COMMENTS

Appointments: ....

Health Concerns: ....

Plans For Tommorow: ....

Pain Level: .... Happiness Level: .... Alertness Level: ....

Supplies Needed Soon: ....

Medication Taken: ....

NOTES

Caregiving Notes For: _____   **Date:** ____ / ____ / ____

	Time							
Toileting	U							
	BM							

Times up During The Night				

Breakfast	
AM Snack	
Lunch	
PM Snack	
Dinner	
Drinks	

ACTIVITIES & OTHER COMMENTS

Appointments: _____

Health Concerns: _____

Plans For Tommorow: _____

Pain Level: _____   Happiness Level: _____   Alertness Level: _____

Supplies Needed Soon: _____

Medication Taken: _____

NOTES

Caregiving Notes For: _____   **Date:** _____ / _____ / _____

Toileting	Time							
	U							
	BM							

Times up During The Night				

Breakfast	
AM Snack	
Lunch	
PM Snack	
Dinner	
Drinks	

ACTIVITIES & OTHER COMMENTS

Appointments: _____

Health Concerns: _____

Plans For Tommorow: _____

Pain Level: _____ Happiness Level: _____ Alertness Level: _____

Supplies Needed Soon: _____

Medication Taken: _____

NOTES

Caregiving Notes For: _____   **Date:** _____ / _____ / _____

Toileting	Time						
	U						
	BM						

Times up During The Night			

Breakfast	
AM Snack	
Lunch	
PM Snack	
Dinner	
Drinks	

ACTIVITIES & OTHER COMMENTS

Appointments: _____

Health Concerns: _____

Plans For Tommorow: _____

Pain Level: _____ Happiness Level: _____ Alertness Level: _____

Supplies Needed Soon: _____

Medication Taken: _____

NOTES

Caregiving Notes For: _____ **Date:** _____ / _____ / _____

Toileting								
	Time							
	U							
	BM							

Times up During The Night				

Breakfast	
AM Snack	
Lunch	
PM Snack	
Dinner	
Drinks	

ACTIVITIES & OTHER COMMENTS

Appointments: _____

Health Concerns: _____

Plans For Tommorow: _____

Pain Level: _____ Happiness Level: _____ Alertness Level: _____

Supplies Needed Soon: _____

Medication Taken: _____

NOTES

Caregiving Notes For: _____   **Date:** ____ / ____ / ____

Toileting								
	Time							
	U							
	BM							

Times up During The Night			

Breakfast	
AM Snack	
Lunch	
PM Snack	
Dinner	
Drinks	

ACTIVITIES & OTHER COMMENTS

Appointments: _____

Health Concerns: _____

Plans For Tommorow: _____

Pain Level: _____ Happiness Level: _____ Alertness Level: _____

Supplies Needed Soon: _____

Medication Taken: _____

NOTES

Caregiving Notes For: _____   **Date:** ____ / ____ / ____

Toileting	Time							
	U							
	BM							

Times up During The Night				

Breakfast	
AM Snack	
Lunch	
PM Snack	
Dinner	
Drinks	

ACTIVITIES & OTHER COMMENTS

Appointments: _____

Health Concerns: _____

Plans For Tommorow: _____

Pain Level: _____ Happiness Level: _____ Alertness Level: _____

Supplies Needed Soon: _____

Medication Taken: _____

NOTES

Caregiving Notes For: _____ **Date:** _____ / _____ / _____

Toileting	Time							
	U							
	BM							

Times up During The Night			

Breakfast	
AM Snack	
Lunch	
PM Snack	
Dinner	
Drinks	

ACTIVITIES & OTHER COMMENTS

Appointments: _____

Health Concerns: _____

Plans For Tommorow: _____

Pain Level:_____ Happiness Level:_____ Alertness Level:_____

Supplies Needed Soon: _____

Medication Taken:_____

NOTES

Caregiving Notes For: _____   **Date:** _____ / _____ / _____

	Time						
Toileting	U						
	BM						

Times up During The Night				

Breakfast	
AM Snack	
Lunch	
PM Snack	
Dinner	
Drinks	

ACTIVITIES & OTHER COMMENTS

Appointments: _____

Health Concerns: _____

Plans For Tommorow: _____

Pain Level: _____   Happiness Level: _____   Alertness Level: _____

Supplies Needed Soon: _____

Medication Taken: _____

NOTES

Caregiving Notes For: _____   **Date:** _____ / _____ / _____

Toileting	Time						
	U						
	BM						

Times up During The Night			

Breakfast	
AM Snack	
Lunch	
PM Snack	
Dinner	
Drinks	

ACTIVITIES & OTHER COMMENTS

Appointments: _____

Health Concerns: _____

Plans For Tommorow: _____

Pain Level: _____ Happiness Level: _____ Alertness Level: _____

Supplies Needed Soon: _____

Medication Taken: _____

NOTES

Caregiving Notes For: ....   **Date:** ——— / ——— / ———

Toileting	Time							
	U							
	BM							

Times up During The Night				

Breakfast	
AM Snack	
Lunch	
PM Snack	
Dinner	
Drinks	

ACTIVITIES & OTHER COMMENTS

Appointments: ....

Health Concerns: ....

Plans For Tommorow: ....

Pain Level: .... Happiness Level: .... Alertness Level: ....

Supplies Needed Soon: ....

Medication Taken: ....

NOTES

Caregiving Notes For: _____   Date: ____ / ____ / ____

Toileting							
	Time						
	U						
	BM						

Times up During The Night				

Breakfast	
AM Snack	
Lunch	
PM Snack	
Dinner	
Drinks	

ACTIVITIES & OTHER COMMENTS

Appointments: _____

Health Concerns: _____

Plans For Tommorow: _____

Pain Level: _____ Happiness Level: _____ Alertness Level: _____

Supplies Needed Soon: _____

Medication Taken: _____

NOTES

Caregiving Notes For: _____ **Date:** _____ / _____ / _____

Toileting	Time						
	U						
	BM						

Times up During The Night | | | | |

Breakfast	
AM Snack	
Lunch	
PM Snack	
Dinner	
Drinks	

ACTIVITIES & OTHER COMMENTS

_____
_____
_____
_____
_____

Appointments: _____

Health Concerns: _____

Plans For Tommorow: _____

Pain Level: _____ Happiness Level: _____ Alertness Level: _____

Supplies Needed Soon: _____

Medication Taken: _____

NOTES

_____
_____
_____
_____

Caregiving Notes For: _____ **Date:** ____ / ____ / ____

Toileting	Time						
	U						
	BM						

Times up During The Night				

Breakfast	
AM Snack	
Lunch	
PM Snack	
Dinner	
Drinks	

ACTIVITIES & OTHER COMMENTS

Appointments: _____

Health Concerns: _____

Plans For Tommorow: _____

Pain Level: _____ Happiness Level: _____ Alertness Level: _____

Supplies Needed Soon: _____

Medication Taken: _____

NOTES

Caregiving Notes For: .... **Date:** ——— / ——— / ———

Toileting								
	Time							
	U							
	BM							

Times up During The Night				

Breakfast	
AM Snack	
Lunch	
PM Snack	
Dinner	
Drinks	

ACTIVITIES & OTHER COMMENTS

Appointments: ....

Health Concerns: ....

Plans For Tommorow: ....

Pain Level: .... Happiness Level: .... Alertness Level: ....

Supplies Needed Soon: ....

Medication Taken: ....

NOTES

Caregiving Notes For: _____   **Date:** _____ / _____ / _____

<table>
<tr><td rowspan="3">Toileting</td><td>Time</td><td></td><td></td><td></td><td></td><td></td><td></td></tr>
<tr><td>U</td><td></td><td></td><td></td><td></td><td></td><td></td></tr>
<tr><td>BM</td><td></td><td></td><td></td><td></td><td></td><td></td></tr>
</table>

Times up During The Night				

Breakfast	
AM Snack	
Lunch	
PM Snack	
Dinner	
Drinks	

ACTIVITIES & OTHER COMMENTS

_____

_____

_____

_____

Appointments: _____

Health Concerns: _____

Plans For Tommorow: _____

Pain Level: _____ Happiness Level: _____ Alertness Level: _____

Supplies Needed Soon: _____

Medication Taken: _____

NOTES

_____

_____

_____

_____

Caregiving Notes For: .... **Date:** _____ / _____ / _____

Toileting	Time							
	U							
	BM							

Times up During The Night				

Breakfast	
AM Snack	
Lunch	
PM Snack	
Dinner	
Drinks	

ACTIVITIES & OTHER COMMENTS

Appointments: ....

Health Concerns: ....

Plans For Tommorow: ....

Pain Level: .... Happiness Level: .... Alertness Level: ....

Supplies Needed Soon: ....

Medication Taken: ....

NOTES

Caregiving Notes For: _____ **Date:** ____ / ____ / ____

Toileting	Time							
	U							
	BM							

Times up During The Night				

Breakfast	
AM Snack	
Lunch	
PM Snack	
Dinner	
Drinks	

ACTIVITIES & OTHER COMMENTS

Appointments: _____

Health Concerns: _____

Plans For Tommorow: _____

Pain Level: _____ Happiness Level: _____ Alertness Level: _____

Supplies Needed Soon: _____

Medication Taken: _____

NOTES

Caregiving Notes For: .... **Date:** _____ / _____ / _____

Toileting									
	Time								
	U								
	BM								

Times up During The Night				

Breakfast	
AM Snack	
Lunch	
PM Snack	
Dinner	
Drinks	

ACTIVITIES & OTHER COMMENTS

Appointments: ....

Health Concerns: ....

Plans For Tommorow: ....

Pain Level:.......................... Happiness Level:.......................... Alertness Level:..........................

Supplies Needed Soon: ....

Medication Taken:...

NOTES

Caregiving Notes For: _____ **Date:** _____ / _____ / _____

Toileting	Time							
	U							
	BM							

Times up During The Night				

Breakfast	
AM Snack	
Lunch	
PM Snack	
Dinner	
Drinks	

ACTIVITIES & OTHER COMMENTS

Appointments: _____

Health Concerns: _____

Plans For Tommorow: _____

Pain Level: _____ Happiness Level: _____ Alertness Level: _____

Supplies Needed Soon: _____

Medication Taken: _____

NOTES

Caregiving Notes For: _____ **Date:** _____ / _____ / _____

Toileting	Time							
	U							
	BM							

Times up During The Night				

Breakfast	
AM Snack	
Lunch	
PM Snack	
Dinner	
Drinks	

ACTIVITIES & OTHER COMMENTS

_____
_____
_____
_____
_____

Appointments: _____

Health Concerns: _____

Plans For Tommorow: _____

Pain Level: _____ Happiness Level: _____ Alertness Level: _____

Supplies Needed Soon: _____

Medication Taken: _____

NOTES

_____
_____
_____
_____

Caregiving Notes For: _____ **Date:** _____ / _____ / _____

Toileting	Time						
	U						
	BM						

Times up During The Night				

Breakfast	
AM Snack	
Lunch	
PM Snack	
Dinner	
Drinks	

ACTIVITIES & OTHER COMMENTS

Appointments: _____

Health Concerns: _____

Plans For Tommorow: _____

Pain Level: _____ Happiness Level: _____ Alertness Level: _____

Supplies Needed Soon: _____

Medication Taken: _____

NOTES

Caregiving Notes For: _____ **Date:** ____ / ____ / ____

Toileting								
	Time							
	U							
	BM							

Times up During The Night				

Breakfast	
AM Snack	
Lunch	
PM Snack	
Dinner	
Drinks	

ACTIVITIES & OTHER COMMENTS

Appointments: _____

Health Concerns: _____

Plans For Tommorow: _____

Pain Level: _____ Happiness Level: _____ Alertness Level: _____

Supplies Needed Soon: _____

Medication Taken: _____

NOTES

Caregiving Notes For: .... **Date:** .... / .... / ....

Toileting	Time						
	U						
	BM						

Times up During The Night				

Breakfast	
AM Snack	
Lunch	
PM Snack	
Dinner	
Drinks	

ACTIVITIES & OTHER COMMENTS

Appointments: ....

Health Concerns: ....

Plans For Tommorow: ....

Pain Level: .... Happiness Level: .... Alertness Level: ....

Supplies Needed Soon: ....

Medication Taken: ....

NOTES

Caregiving Notes For: _____ **Date:** _____ / _____ / _____

Toileting	Time							
	U							
	BM							

Times up During The Night				

Breakfast	
AM Snack	
Lunch	
PM Snack	
Dinner	
Drinks	

ACTIVITIES & OTHER COMMENTS

Appointments: _____

Health Concerns: _____

Plans For Tommorow: _____

Pain Level: _____ Happiness Level: _____ Alertness Level: _____

Supplies Needed Soon: _____

Medication Taken: _____

NOTES

Caregiving Notes For: _____ **Date:** _____ / _____ / _____

Toileting								
	Time							
	U							
	BM							

Times up During The Night				

Breakfast	
AM Snack	
Lunch	
PM Snack	
Dinner	
Drinks	

ACTIVITIES & OTHER COMMENTS

Appointments: _____

Health Concerns: _____

Plans For Tommorow: _____

Pain Level: _____ Happiness Level: _____ Alertness Level: _____

Supplies Needed Soon: _____

Medication Taken: _____

NOTES

Caregiving Notes For: _____ **Date:** _____ / _____ / _____

Toileting								
	Time							
	U							
	BM							

Times up During The Night				

Breakfast	
AM Snack	
Lunch	
PM Snack	
Dinner	
Drinks	

ACTIVITIES & OTHER COMMENTS

Appointments: _____

Health Concerns: _____

Plans For Tommorow: _____

Pain Level: _____ Happiness Level: _____ Alertness Level: _____

Supplies Needed Soon: _____

Medication Taken: _____

NOTES

Caregiving Notes For: _____ **Date:** _____ / _____ / _____

Toileting	Time							
	U							
	BM							

Times up During The Night				

Breakfast	
AM Snack	
Lunch	
PM Snack	
Dinner	
Drinks	

ACTIVITIES & OTHER COMMENTS

Appointments: _____

Health Concerns: _____

Plans For Tommorow: _____

Pain Level: _____ Happiness Level: _____ Alertness Level: _____

Supplies Needed Soon: _____

Medication Taken: _____

NOTES

Caregiving Notes For: _____ **Date:** _____ / _____ / _____

Toileting	Time							
	U							
	BM							

Times up During The Night				

Breakfast	
AM Snack	
Lunch	
PM Snack	
Dinner	
Drinks	

ACTIVITIES & OTHER COMMENTS

Appointments: _____

Health Concerns: _____

Plans For Tommorow: _____

Pain Level: _____ Happiness Level: _____ Alertness Level: _____

Supplies Needed Soon: _____

Medication Taken: _____

NOTES

Caregiving Notes For: _____ **Date:** _____ / _____ / _____

Toileting	Time							
	U							
	BM							

Times up During The Night			

Breakfast	
AM Snack	
Lunch	
PM Snack	
Dinner	
Drinks	

ACTIVITIES & OTHER COMMENTS

Appointments: _____

Health Concerns: _____

Plans For Tommorow: _____

Pain Level: _____ Happiness Level: _____ Alertness Level: _____

Supplies Needed Soon: _____

Medication Taken: _____

NOTES

Caregiving Notes For: _____ **Date:** _____ / _____ / _____

Toileting	Time							
	U							
	BM							

Times up During The Night				

Breakfast	
AM Snack	
Lunch	
PM Snack	
Dinner	
Drinks	

ACTIVITIES & OTHER COMMENTS

Appointments: _____

Health Concerns: _____

Plans For Tommorow: _____

Pain Level: _____ Happiness Level: _____ Alertness Level: _____

Supplies Needed Soon: _____

Medication Taken: _____

NOTES

Caregiving Notes For: _____ **Date:** ____ / ____ / ____

Toileting	Time							
	U							
	BM							

Times up During The Night				

Breakfast	
AM Snack	
Lunch	
PM Snack	
Dinner	
Drinks	

ACTIVITIES & OTHER COMMENTS

Appointments: _____

Health Concerns: _____

Plans For Tommorow: _____

Pain Level: _____ Happiness Level: _____ Alertness Level: _____

Supplies Needed Soon: _____

Medication Taken: _____

NOTES

Caregiving Notes For: _____ **Date:** ____ / ____ / ____

Toileting	Time							
	U							
	BM							

Times up During The Night				

Breakfast	
AM Snack	
Lunch	
PM Snack	
Dinner	
Drinks	

ACTIVITIES & OTHER COMMENTS

Appointments: _____

Health Concerns: _____

Plans For Tommorow: _____

Pain Level: _____ Happiness Level: _____ Alertness Level: _____

Supplies Needed Soon: _____

Medication Taken: _____

NOTES

Caregiving Notes For: _____ **Date:** _____ / _____ / _____

Toileting	Time						
	U						
	BM						

Times up During The Night				

Breakfast	
AM Snack	
Lunch	
PM Snack	
Dinner	
Drinks	

ACTIVITIES & OTHER COMMENTS

Appointments: _____

Health Concerns: _____

Plans For Tommorow: _____

Pain Level: _____ Happiness Level: _____ Alertness Level: _____

Supplies Needed Soon: _____

Medication Taken: _____

NOTES

Caregiving Notes For: _____   **Date:** ____ / ____ / ____

Toileting	Time							
	U							
	BM							

Times up During The Night				

Breakfast	
AM Snack	
Lunch	
PM Snack	
Dinner	
Drinks	

ACTIVITIES & OTHER COMMENTS

Appointments: _____

Health Concerns: _____

Plans For Tommorow: _____

Pain Level: _____ Happiness Level: _____ Alertness Level: _____

Supplies Needed Soon: _____

Medication Taken: _____

NOTES

Caregiving Notes For: _____ **Date:** _____ / _____ / _____

Toileting	Time						
	U						
	BM						

Times up During The Night				

Breakfast	
AM Snack	
Lunch	
PM Snack	
Dinner	
Drinks	

ACTIVITIES & OTHER COMMENTS

Appointments: _____

Health Concerns: _____

Plans For Tommorow: _____

Pain Level: _____ Happiness Level: _____ Alertness Level: _____

Supplies Needed Soon: _____

Medication Taken: _____

NOTES

Caregiving Notes For: .... **Date:** .... / .... / ....

<table>
<tr><td rowspan="3">Toileting</td><td>Time</td><td></td><td></td><td></td><td></td><td></td><td></td></tr>
<tr><td>U</td><td></td><td></td><td></td><td></td><td></td><td></td></tr>
<tr><td>BM</td><td></td><td></td><td></td><td></td><td></td><td></td></tr>
</table>

Times up During The Night				

Breakfast	
AM Snack	
Lunch	
PM Snack	
Dinner	
Drinks	

ACTIVITIES & OTHER COMMENTS

Appointments: ....

Health Concerns: ....

Plans For Tommorow: ....

Pain Level: .... Happiness Level: .... Alertness Level: ....

Supplies Needed Soon: ....

Medication Taken: ....

NOTES

Caregiving Notes For: .... **Date:** .... / .... / ....

		Time							
Toileting		U							
		BM							

Times up During The Night			

Breakfast	
AM Snack	
Lunch	
PM Snack	
Dinner	
Drinks	

ACTIVITIES & OTHER COMMENTS

Appointments: ....

Health Concerns: ....

Plans For Tommorow: ....

Pain Level: .... Happiness Level: .... Alertness Level: ....

Supplies Needed Soon: ....

Medication Taken: ....

NOTES

Caregiving Notes For: _____ **Date:** _____ / _____ /

Toileting	Time							
	U							
	BM							

Times up During The Night				

Breakfast	
AM Snack	
Lunch	
PM Snack	
Dinner	
Drinks	

ACTIVITIES & OTHER COMMENTS

Appointments: _____

Health Concerns: _____

Plans For Tommorow: _____

Pain Level: _____ Happiness Level: _____ Alertness Level: _____

Supplies Needed Soon: _____

Medication Taken: _____

NOTES

Caregiving Notes For: _____ **Date:** _____ / _____ / _____

Toileting								
	Time							
	U							
	BM							

Times up During The Night				

Breakfast	
AM Snack	
Lunch	
PM Snack	
Dinner	
Drinks	

ACTIVITIES & OTHER COMMENTS

Appointments: _____

Health Concerns: _____

Plans For Tommorow: _____

Pain Level: _____ Happiness Level: _____ Alertness Level: _____

Supplies Needed Soon: _____

Medication Taken: _____

NOTES

Caregiving Notes For: .... **Date:** .... / .... / ....

Toileting	Time						
	U						
	BM						

Times up During The Night			

Breakfast	
AM Snack	
Lunch	
PM Snack	
Dinner	
Drinks	

ACTIVITIES & OTHER COMMENTS

Appointments: ....

Health Concerns: ....

Plans For Tommorow: ....

Pain Level:................... Happiness Level:.................. Alertness Level:...........

Supplies Needed Soon: ....

Medication Taken:..

NOTES

Caregiving Notes For: _____   **Date:** ___ / ___ / ___

Toileting	Time							
	U							
	BM							

Times up During The Night				

Breakfast	
AM Snack	
Lunch	
PM Snack	
Dinner	
Drinks	

ACTIVITIES & OTHER COMMENTS

Appointments: _____

Health Concerns: _____

Plans For Tommorow: _____

Pain Level: _____   Happiness Level: _____   Alertness Level: _____

Supplies Needed Soon: _____

Medication Taken: _____

NOTES

Caregiving Notes For: .... **Date:** _____ / _____ / _____

Toileting	Time							
	U							
	BM							

Times up During The Night				

Breakfast	
AM Snack	
Lunch	
PM Snack	
Dinner	
Drinks	

ACTIVITIES & OTHER COMMENTS

Appointments: ....

Health Concerns: ....

Plans For Tommorow: ....

Pain Level: .... Happiness Level: .... Alertness Level: ....

Supplies Needed Soon: ....

Medication Taken: ....

NOTES

Caregiving Notes For: .... **Date:** _____ / _____ / _____

Toileting	Time							
	U							
	BM							

Times up During The Night

Breakfast	
AM Snack	
Lunch	
PM Snack	
Dinner	
Drinks	

ACTIVITIES & OTHER COMMENTS

Appointments: ....

Health Concerns: ....

Plans For Tommorow: ....

Pain Level:..................... Happiness Level:..................... Alertness Level:.....................

Supplies Needed Soon: ....

Medication Taken:..

NOTES

Caregiving Notes For: .... **Date:** .... / .... / ....

Toileting	Time							
	U							
	BM							

Times up During The Night			

Breakfast	
AM Snack	
Lunch	
PM Snack	
Dinner	
Drinks	

ACTIVITIES & OTHER COMMENTS

Appointments: ....

Health Concerns: ....

Plans For Tommorow: ....

Pain Level: .... Happiness Level: .... Alertness Level: ....

Supplies Needed Soon: ....

Medication Taken: ....

NOTES

Caregiving Notes For: _____   **Date:** _____ / _____ / _____

Toileting	Time							
	U							
	BM							

Times up During The Night				

Breakfast	
AM Snack	
Lunch	
PM Snack	
Dinner	
Drinks	

ACTIVITIES & OTHER COMMENTS

Appointments: _____

Health Concerns: _____

Plans For Tommorow: _____

Pain Level: _____ Happiness Level: _____ Alertness Level: _____

Supplies Needed Soon: _____

Medication Taken: _____

NOTES

Caregiving Notes For: _____ **Date:** ____ / ____ / ____

	Time						
Toileting	U						
	BM						

Times up During The Night				

Breakfast	
AM Snack	
Lunch	
PM Snack	
Dinner	
Drinks	

ACTIVITIES & OTHER COMMENTS

Appointments: _____

Health Concerns: _____

Plans For Tommorow: _____

Pain Level: _____ Happiness Level: _____ Alertness Level: _____

Supplies Needed Soon: _____

Medication Taken: _____

NOTES

Caregiving Notes For: .... **Date:** .... / .... / ....

Toileting	Time							
	U							
	BM							

Times up During The Night				

Breakfast	
AM Snack	
Lunch	
PM Snack	
Dinner	
Drinks	

ACTIVITIES & OTHER COMMENTS

Appointments: ....

Health Concerns: ....

Plans For Tommorow: ....

Pain Level: .... Happiness Level: .... Alertness Level: ....

Supplies Needed Soon: ....

Medication Taken: ....

NOTES

Caregiving Notes For: _____   **Date:** _____ / _____ / _____

Toileting	Time						
	U						
	BM						

Times up During The Night				

Breakfast	
AM Snack	
Lunch	
PM Snack	
Dinner	
Drinks	

ACTIVITIES & OTHER COMMENTS

Appointments: _____

Health Concerns: _____

Plans For Tommorow: _____

Pain Level: _____ Happiness Level: _____ Alertness Level: _____

Supplies Needed Soon: _____

Medication Taken: _____

NOTES

Caregiving Notes For: _____ **Date:** _____ / _____ / _____

Toileting	Time							
	U							
	BM							

Times up During The Night				

Breakfast	
AM Snack	
Lunch	
PM Snack	
Dinner	
Drinks	

ACTIVITIES & OTHER COMMENTS

Appointments: _____

Health Concerns: _____

Plans For Tommorow: _____

Pain Level: _____ Happiness Level: _____ Alertness Level: _____

Supplies Needed Soon: _____

Medication Taken: _____

NOTES

Caregiving Notes For: _____ **Date:** _____ / _____ / _____

Toileting								
	Time							
	U							
	BM							

Times up During The Night				

Breakfast	
AM Snack	
Lunch	
PM Snack	
Dinner	
Drinks	

ACTIVITIES & OTHER COMMENTS

Appointments: _____

Health Concerns: _____

Plans For Tommorow: _____

Pain Level: _____ Happiness Level: _____ Alertness Level: _____

Supplies Needed Soon: _____

Medication Taken: _____

NOTES

Caregiving Notes For: ....   **Date:** ..../......../........

Toileting	Time							
	U							
	BM							

Times up During The Night				

Breakfast	
AM Snack	
Lunch	
PM Snack	
Dinner	
Drinks	

ACTIVITIES & OTHER COMMENTS

Appointments: ....

Health Concerns: ....

Plans For Tommorow: ....

Pain Level: .... Happiness Level: .... Alertness Level: ....

Supplies Needed Soon: ....

Medication Taken: ....

NOTES

Caregiving Notes For: .... **Date:** _____ / _____ / _____

<table>
<tr><td rowspan="3">Toileting</td><td>Time</td><td></td><td></td><td></td><td></td><td></td><td></td></tr>
<tr><td>U</td><td></td><td></td><td></td><td></td><td></td><td></td></tr>
<tr><td>BM</td><td></td><td></td><td></td><td></td><td></td><td></td></tr>
</table>

Times up During The Night				

Breakfast	
AM Snack	
Lunch	
PM Snack	
Dinner	
Drinks	

ACTIVITIES & OTHER COMMENTS

Appointments: ....

Health Concerns: ....

Plans For Tommorow: ....

Pain Level: .... Happiness Level: .... Alertness Level: ....

Supplies Needed Soon: ....

Medication Taken: ....

NOTES

Caregiving Notes For: _____ **Date:** ____ / ____ / ____

Toileting	Time							
	U							
	BM							

Times up During The Night				

Breakfast	
AM Snack	
Lunch	
PM Snack	
Dinner	
Drinks	

ACTIVITIES & OTHER COMMENTS

Appointments: _____

Health Concerns: _____

Plans For Tommorow: _____

Pain Level: _____ Happiness Level: _____ Alertness Level: _____

Supplies Needed Soon: _____

Medication Taken: _____

NOTES

Caregiving Notes For: _____ **Date:** _____ / _____ / _____

Toileting								
	Time							
	U							
	BM							

Times up During The Night				

Breakfast	
AM Snack	
Lunch	
PM Snack	
Dinner	
Drinks	

ACTIVITIES & OTHER COMMENTS

Appointments: _____

Health Concerns: _____

Plans For Tommorow: _____

Pain Level: _____ Happiness Level: _____ Alertness Level: _____

Supplies Needed Soon: _____

Medication Taken: _____

NOTES

Caregiving Notes For: _____ **Date:** ____ / ____ / ____

Toileting	Time						
	U						
	BM						

Times up During The Night				

Breakfast	
AM Snack	
Lunch	
PM Snack	
Dinner	
Drinks	

ACTIVITIES & OTHER COMMENTS

Appointments: _____

Health Concerns: _____

Plans For Tommorow: _____

Pain Level: _____ Happiness Level: _____ Alertness Level: _____

Supplies Needed Soon: _____

Medication Taken: _____

NOTES

Caregiving Notes For: _____ **Date:** ____ / ____ / ____

Toileting	Time						
	U						
	BM						

Times up During The Night				

Breakfast	
AM Snack	
Lunch	
PM Snack	
Dinner	
Drinks	

ACTIVITIES & OTHER COMMENTS

Appointments: _____

Health Concerns: _____

Plans For Tommorow: _____

Pain Level: _____ Happiness Level: _____ Alertness Level: _____

Supplies Needed Soon: _____

Medication Taken: _____

NOTES

Caregiving Notes For: .... **Date:** .... / .... / ....

Toileting	Time							
	U							
	BM							

Times up During The Night				

Breakfast	
AM Snack	
Lunch	
PM Snack	
Dinner	
Drinks	

ACTIVITIES & OTHER COMMENTS

Appointments: --

Health Concerns: --

Plans For Tommorow: ---

Pain Level: ------------ Happiness Level: ------------ Alertness Level: ------------

Supplies Needed Soon: ---

Medication Taken: --

NOTES

Caregiving Notes For: _____ **Date:** _____ / _____ / _____

Toileting	Time						
	U						
	BM						

Times up During The Night				

Breakfast	
AM Snack	
Lunch	
PM Snack	
Dinner	
Drinks	

ACTIVITIES & OTHER COMMENTS

Appointments: _____

Health Concerns: _____

Plans For Tommorow: _____

Pain Level: _____ Happiness Level: _____ Alertness Level: _____

Supplies Needed Soon: _____

Medication Taken: _____

NOTES

Caregiving Notes For: _____ **Date:** ____ / ____ / ____

Toileting	Time							
	U							
	BM							

Times up During The Night					

Breakfast	
AM Snack	
Lunch	
PM Snack	
Dinner	
Drinks	

ACTIVITIES & OTHER COMMENTS

_____
_____
_____
_____
_____

Appointments: _____

Health Concerns: _____

Plans For Tommorow: _____

Pain Level: _____ Happiness Level: _____ Alertness Level: _____

Supplies Needed Soon: _____

Medication Taken: _____

NOTES

_____
_____
_____
_____
_____

Caregiving Notes For: _____ **Date:** ____ / ____ / ____

Toileting							
	Time						
	U						
	BM						

Times up During The Night				

Breakfast	
AM Snack	
Lunch	
PM Snack	
Dinner	
Drinks	

ACTIVITIES & OTHER COMMENTS

_____
_____
_____
_____
_____

Appointments: _____

Health Concerns: _____

Plans For Tommorow: _____

Pain Level: _____ Happiness Level: _____ Alertness Level: _____

Supplies Needed Soon: _____

Medication Taken: _____

NOTES

_____
_____
_____
_____

Caregiving Notes For: _____ **Date:** ____ / ____ / ____

Toileting	Time							
	U							
	BM							

Times up During The Night				

Breakfast	
AM Snack	
Lunch	
PM Snack	
Dinner	
Drinks	

ACTIVITIES & OTHER COMMENTS

Appointments: _____

Health Concerns: _____

Plans For Tommorow: _____

Pain Level: _____ Happiness Level: _____ Alertness Level: _____

Supplies Needed Soon: _____

Medication Taken: _____

NOTES

Caregiving Notes For: _____ **Date:** _____ / _____ / _____

Toileting	Time							
	U							
	BM							

Times up During The Night				

Breakfast	
AM Snack	
Lunch	
PM Snack	
Dinner	
Drinks	

ACTIVITIES & OTHER COMMENTS

Appointments: _____

Health Concerns: _____

Plans For Tommorow: _____

Pain Level: _____ Happiness Level: _____ Alertness Level: _____

Supplies Needed Soon: _____

Medication Taken: _____

NOTES

Caregiving Notes For: .... **Date:** .... / .... / ....

Toileting	Time						
	U						
	BM						

Times up During The Night			

Breakfast	
AM Snack	
Lunch	
PM Snack	
Dinner	
Drinks	

ACTIVITIES & OTHER COMMENTS

Appointments: ....

Health Concerns: ....

Plans For Tommorow: ....

Pain Level:.................................... Happiness Level:............................. Alertness Level:...................

Supplies Needed Soon: ....

Medication Taken:...

NOTES

Caregiving Notes For: _____ **Date:** _____ / _____ / _____

Toileting	Time							
	U							
	BM							

Times up During The Night				

Breakfast	
AM Snack	
Lunch	
PM Snack	
Dinner	
Drinks	

ACTIVITIES & OTHER COMMENTS

Appointments: _____

Health Concerns: _____

Plans For Tommorow: _____

Pain Level: _____ Happiness Level: _____ Alertness Level: _____

Supplies Needed Soon: _____

Medication Taken: _____

NOTES

Caregiving Notes For: _____ **Date:** ____ / ____ / ____

Toileting									
	Time								
	U								
	BM								

Times up During The Night				

Breakfast	
AM Snack	
Lunch	
PM Snack	
Dinner	
Drinks	

ACTIVITIES & OTHER COMMENTS

Appointments: _____

Health Concerns: _____

Plans For Tommorow: _____

Pain Level: _____ Happiness Level: _____ Alertness Level: _____

Supplies Needed Soon: _____

Medication Taken: _____

NOTES

Caregiving Notes For: _____ **Date:** _____ / _____ / _____

	Toileting							
	Time							
	U							
	BM							

Times up During The Night | | | | |

Breakfast	
AM Snack	
Lunch	
PM Snack	
Dinner	
Drinks	

ACTIVITIES & OTHER COMMENTS

Appointments: _____

Health Concerns: _____

Plans For Tommorow: _____

Pain Level: _____ Happiness Level: _____ Alertness Level: _____

Supplies Needed Soon: _____

Medication Taken: _____

NOTES

Caregiving Notes For: _____ Date: ____ / ____ / ____

Toileting	Time						
	U						
	BM						

Times up During The Night				

Breakfast	
AM Snack	
Lunch	
PM Snack	
Dinner	
Drinks	

ACTIVITIES & OTHER COMMENTS

Appointments: _____

Health Concerns: _____

Plans For Tommorow: _____

Pain Level: _____ Happiness Level: _____ Alertness Level: _____

Supplies Needed Soon: _____

Medication Taken: _____

NOTES

Caregiving Notes For: _____   **Date:** _____ / _____ / _____

Toileting	Time							
	U							
	BM							

Times up During The Night				

Breakfast	
AM Snack	
Lunch	
PM Snack	
Dinner	
Drinks	

ACTIVITIES & OTHER COMMENTS

Appointments: _____

Health Concerns: _____

Plans For Tommorow: _____

Pain Level: _____ Happiness Level: _____ Alertness Level: _____

Supplies Needed Soon: _____

Medication Taken: _____

NOTES

Caregiving Notes For: .... **Date:** ...... / ...... / ......

Toileting							
	Time						
	U						
	BM						

Times up During The Night				

Breakfast	
AM Snack	
Lunch	
PM Snack	
Dinner	
Drinks	

ACTIVITIES & OTHER COMMENTS

Appointments: ....

Health Concerns: ....

Plans For Tommorow: ....

Pain Level: .... Happiness Level: .... Alertness Level: ....

Supplies Needed Soon: ....

Medication Taken: ....

NOTES

Caregiving Notes For: _____ **Date:** ____/____/____

Toileting	Time						
	U						
	BM						

Times up During The Night				

Breakfast	
AM Snack	
Lunch	
PM Snack	
Dinner	
Drinks	

ACTIVITIES & OTHER COMMENTS

Appointments: _____

Health Concerns: _____

Plans For Tommorow: _____

Pain Level: _____ Happiness Level: _____ Alertness Level: _____

Supplies Needed Soon: _____

Medication Taken: _____

NOTES

Caregiving Notes For: _____ **Date:** ____ / ____ / ____

Toileting	Time							
	U							
	BM							

Times up During The Night				

Breakfast	
AM Snack	
Lunch	
PM Snack	
Dinner	
Drinks	

ACTIVITIES & OTHER COMMENTS

Appointments: _____

Health Concerns: _____

Plans For Tommorow: _____

Pain Level: _____ Happiness Level: _____ Alertness Level: _____

Supplies Needed Soon: _____

Medication Taken: _____

NOTES

Caregiving Notes For: _____   **Date:** _____ / _____ / _____

Toileting								
	Time							
	U							
	BM							

Times up During The Night				

Breakfast	
AM Snack	
Lunch	
PM Snack	
Dinner	
Drinks	

ACTIVITIES & OTHER COMMENTS

Appointments: _____

Health Concerns: _____

Plans For Tommorow: _____

Pain Level: _____ Happiness Level: _____ Alertness Level: _____

Supplies Needed Soon: _____

Medication Taken: _____

NOTES

Caregiving Notes For: _____   **Date:** ____ / ____ / ____

Toileting	Time						
	U						
	BM						

Times up During The Night				

Breakfast	
AM Snack	
Lunch	
PM Snack	
Dinner	
Drinks	

ACTIVITIES & OTHER COMMENTS

Appointments: _____

Health Concerns: _____

Plans For Tommorow: _____

Pain Level: _____ Happiness Level: _____ Alertness Level: _____

Supplies Needed Soon: _____

Medication Taken: _____

NOTES

Caregiving Notes For: _____   Date: _____ / _____ / _____

Toileting	Time							
	U							
	BM							

Times up During The Night				

Breakfast	
AM Snack	
Lunch	
PM Snack	
Dinner	
Drinks	

ACTIVITIES & OTHER COMMENTS

Appointments: _____

Health Concerns: _____

Plans For Tommorow: _____

Pain Level: _____ Happiness Level: _____ Alertness Level: _____

Supplies Needed Soon: _____

Medication Taken: _____

NOTES

Caregiving Notes For: .... **Date:** .... / .... / ....

Toileting	Time							
	U							
	BM							

Times up During The Night				

Breakfast	
AM Snack	
Lunch	
PM Snack	
Dinner	
Drinks	

ACTIVITIES & OTHER COMMENTS

Appointments: ....

Health Concerns: ....

Plans For Tommorow: ....

Pain Level: .... Happiness Level: .... Alertness Level: ....

Supplies Needed Soon: ....

Medication Taken: ....

NOTES

Caregiving Notes For: ....   Date: ..... / ..... / .....

Toileting	Time						
	U						
	BM						

Times up During The Night				

Breakfast	
AM Snack	
Lunch	
PM Snack	
Dinner	
Drinks	

ACTIVITIES & OTHER COMMENTS

Appointments: ....

Health Concerns: ....

Plans For Tommorow: ....

Pain Level: ....   Happiness Level: ....   Alertness Level: ....

Supplies Needed Soon: ....

Medication Taken: ....

NOTES

Caregiving Notes For: _____ **Date:** ___ / ___ / ___

Toileting								
	Time							
	U							
	BM							

Times up During The Night				

Breakfast	
AM Snack	
Lunch	
PM Snack	
Dinner	
Drinks	

ACTIVITIES & OTHER COMMENTS

Appointments: _____

Health Concerns: _____

Plans For Tommorow: _____

Pain Level: _____ Happiness Level: _____ Alertness Level: _____

Supplies Needed Soon: _____

Medication Taken: _____

NOTES

Caregiving Notes For: .... **Date:** .... / .... / ....

Toileting	Time							
	U							
	BM							

Times up During The Night				

Breakfast	
AM Snack	
Lunch	
PM Snack	
Dinner	
Drinks	

ACTIVITIES & OTHER COMMENTS

Appointments: ....

Health Concerns: ....

Plans For Tommorow: ....

Pain Level: .... Happiness Level: .... Alertness Level: ....

Supplies Needed Soon: ....

Medication Taken: ....

NOTES

Caregiving Notes For: _____ **Date:** ____ / ____ / ____

Toileting	Time							
	U							
	BM							

Times up During The Night				

Breakfast	
AM Snack	
Lunch	
PM Snack	
Dinner	
Drinks	

ACTIVITIES & OTHER COMMENTS

Appointments: _____

Health Concerns: _____

Plans For Tommorow: _____

Pain Level: _____ Happiness Level: _____ Alertness Level: _____

Supplies Needed Soon: _____

Medication Taken: _____

NOTES

Caregiving Notes For: _____   **Date:** _____ / _____ / _____

Toileting	Time						
	U						
	BM						

Times up During The Night				

Breakfast	
AM Snack	
Lunch	
PM Snack	
Dinner	
Drinks	

ACTIVITIES & OTHER COMMENTS

....
....
....
....
....

Appointments: ....

Health Concerns: ....

Plans For Tommorow: ....

Pain Level: .... Happiness Level: .... Alertness Level: ....

Supplies Needed Soon: ....

Medication Taken: ....

NOTES

....
....
....
....
....

Caregiving Notes For: _____ **Date:** _____ / _____ / _____

Toileting	Time							
	U							
	BM							

Times up During The Night				

Breakfast	
AM Snack	
Lunch	
PM Snack	
Dinner	
Drinks	

ACTIVITIES & OTHER COMMENTS

_____
_____
_____
_____
_____

Appointments: _____

Health Concerns: _____

Plans For Tommorow: _____

Pain Level: _____ Happiness Level: _____ Alertness Level: _____

Supplies Needed Soon: _____

Medication Taken: _____

NOTES

_____
_____
_____
_____

Caregiving Notes For: _____ **Date:** _____ / _____ / _____

Toileting	Time							
	U							
	BM							

Times up During The Night				

Breakfast	
AM Snack	
Lunch	
PM Snack	
Dinner	
Drinks	

ACTIVITIES & OTHER COMMENTS

Appointments: _____

Health Concerns: _____

Plans For Tommorow: _____

Pain Level: _____ Happiness Level: _____ Alertness Level: _____

Supplies Needed Soon: _____

Medication Taken: _____

NOTES

Caregiving Notes For: .... **Date:** .... / .... / ....

Toileting	Time						
	U						
	BM						

Times up During The Night				

Breakfast	
AM Snack	
Lunch	
PM Snack	
Dinner	
Drinks	

ACTIVITIES & OTHER COMMENTS

Appointments: ....

Health Concerns: ....

Plans For Tommorow: ....

Pain Level: .... Happiness Level: .... Alertness Level: ....

Supplies Needed Soon: ....

Medication Taken: ....

NOTES

Caregiving Notes For: .... **Date:** ..../......../........

Toileting	Time							
	U							
	BM							

Times up During The Night				

Breakfast	
AM Snack	
Lunch	
PM Snack	
Dinner	
Drinks	

ACTIVITIES & OTHER COMMENTS

Appointments: ....

Health Concerns: ....

Plans For Tommorow: ....

Pain Level: .... Happiness Level: .... Alertness Level: ....

Supplies Needed Soon: ....

Medication Taken: ....

NOTES

Caregiving Notes For: _____ **Date:** ____ / ____ / ____

Toileting	Time						
	U						
	BM						

Times up During The Night				

Breakfast	
AM Snack	
Lunch	
PM Snack	
Dinner	
Drinks	

ACTIVITIES & OTHER COMMENTS

Appointments: _____

Health Concerns: _____

Plans For Tommorow: _____

Pain Level: _____ Happiness Level: _____ Alertness Level: _____

Supplies Needed Soon: _____

Medication Taken: _____

NOTES

Caregiving Notes For: .... **Date:** .... / .... / ....

Toileting	Time					
	U					
	BM					

Times up During The Night				

Breakfast	
AM Snack	
Lunch	
PM Snack	
Dinner	
Drinks	

ACTIVITIES & OTHER COMMENTS

Appointments: ....

Health Concerns: ....

Plans For Tommorow: ....

Pain Level: .... Happiness Level: .... Alertness Level: ....

Supplies Needed Soon: ....

Medication Taken: ....

NOTES

Caregiving Notes For: _____   **Date:** _____ / _____ / _____

Toileting								
	Time							
	U							
	BM							

Times up During The Night				

Breakfast	
AM Snack	
Lunch	
PM Snack	
Dinner	
Drinks	

ACTIVITIES & OTHER COMMENTS

Appointments: _____

Health Concerns: _____

Plans For Tommorow: _____

Pain Level: _____ Happiness Level: _____ Alertness Level: _____

Supplies Needed Soon: _____

Medication Taken: _____

NOTES

Caregiving Notes For: _____ **Date:** _____ / _____ / _____

Toileting	Time							
	U							
	BM							

Times up During The Night				

Breakfast	
AM Snack	
Lunch	
PM Snack	
Dinner	
Drinks	

ACTIVITIES & OTHER COMMENTS

Appointments: _____

Health Concerns: _____

Plans For Tommorow: _____

Pain Level: _____ Happiness Level: _____ Alertness Level: _____

Supplies Needed Soon: _____

Medication Taken: _____

NOTES

Caregiving Notes For: _____ **Date:** ____/____/____

Toileting								
	Time							
	U							
	BM							

Times up During The Night				

Breakfast	
AM Snack	
Lunch	
PM Snack	
Dinner	
Drinks	

ACTIVITIES & OTHER COMMENTS

Appointments: _____

Health Concerns: _____

Plans For Tommorow: _____

Pain Level:_____ Happiness Level:_____ Alertness Level:_____

Supplies Needed Soon: _____

Medication Taken:_____

NOTES

Caregiving Notes For: _____ **Date:** _____ / _____ / _____

<table>
<tr><td rowspan="3">Toileting</td><td>Time</td><td></td><td></td><td></td><td></td><td></td><td></td></tr>
<tr><td>U</td><td></td><td></td><td></td><td></td><td></td><td></td></tr>
<tr><td>BM</td><td></td><td></td><td></td><td></td><td></td><td></td></tr>
</table>

Times up During The Night | | | |

Breakfast	
AM Snack	
Lunch	
PM Snack	
Dinner	
Drinks	

ACTIVITIES & OTHER COMMENTS

Appointments: _____

Health Concerns: _____

Plans For Tommorow: _____

Pain Level: _____ Happiness Level: _____ Alertness Level: _____

Supplies Needed Soon: _____

Medication Taken: _____

NOTES

Caregiving Notes For: _____ **Date:** ____ / ____ / ____

Toileting	Time							
	U							
	BM							

Times up During The Night				

Breakfast	
AM Snack	
Lunch	
PM Snack	
Dinner	
Drinks	

ACTIVITIES & OTHER COMMENTS

Appointments: _____

Health Concerns: _____

Plans For Tommorow: _____

Pain Level: _____ Happiness Level: _____ Alertness Level: _____

Supplies Needed Soon: _____

Medication Taken: _____

NOTES

Caregiving Notes For: _____ **Date:** ___ / ___ / ___

Toileting	Time							
	U							
	BM							

Times up During The Night				

Breakfast	
AM Snack	
Lunch	
PM Snack	
Dinner	
Drinks	

ACTIVITIES & OTHER COMMENTS

Appointments: _____

Health Concerns: _____

Plans For Tommorow: _____

Pain Level: _____ Happiness Level: _____ Alertness Level: _____

Supplies Needed Soon: _____

Medication Taken: _____

NOTES

Caregiving Notes For: _____ **Date:** _____ / _____ / _____

Toileting								
	Time							
	U							
	BM							

Times up During The Night				

Breakfast	
AM Snack	
Lunch	
PM Snack	
Dinner	
Drinks	

ACTIVITIES & OTHER COMMENTS

Appointments: _____

Health Concerns: _____

Plans For Tommorow: _____

Pain Level: _____ Happiness Level: _____ Alertness Level: _____

Supplies Needed Soon: _____

Medication Taken: _____

NOTES

Caregiving Notes For: ....   Date: _____ / _____ / _____

Toileting	Time						
	U						
	BM						

Times up During The Night				

Breakfast	
AM Snack	
Lunch	
PM Snack	
Dinner	
Drinks	

ACTIVITIES & OTHER COMMENTS

Appointments: ....

Health Concerns: ....

Plans For Tommorow: ....

Pain Level: .... Happiness Level: .... Alertness Level: ....

Supplies Needed Soon: ....

Medication Taken: ....

NOTES

Caregiving Notes For: _____ **Date:** _____ / _____ / _____

Toileting	Time						
	U						
	BM						

Times up During The Night				

Breakfast	
AM Snack	
Lunch	
PM Snack	
Dinner	
Drinks	

ACTIVITIES & OTHER COMMENTS

Appointments: _____

Health Concerns: _____

Plans For Tommorow: _____

Pain Level: _____ Happiness Level: _____ Alertness Level: _____

Supplies Needed Soon: _____

Medication Taken: _____

NOTES

Caregiving Notes For: _____   **Date:** ____ / ____ / ____

Toileting							
	Time						
	U						
	BM						

Times up During The Night				

Breakfast	
AM Snack	
Lunch	
PM Snack	
Dinner	
Drinks	

ACTIVITIES & OTHER COMMENTS

Appointments: _____

Health Concerns: _____

Plans For Tommorow: _____

Pain Level: _____ Happiness Level: _____ Alertness Level: _____

Supplies Needed Soon: _____

Medication Taken: _____

NOTES

Caregiving Notes For: .... **Date:** .... / .... / ....

Toileting								
	Time							
	U							
	BM							

Times up During The Night				

Breakfast	
AM Snack	
Lunch	
PM Snack	
Dinner	
Drinks	

ACTIVITIES & OTHER COMMENTS

Appointments: ....

Health Concerns: ....

Plans For Tommorow: ....

Pain Level: .... Happiness Level: .... Alertness Level: ....

Supplies Needed Soon: ....

Medication Taken: ....

NOTES

Caregiving Notes For: _____ Date: _____ / _____ / _____

Toileting									
	Time								
	U								
	BM								

Times up During The Night				

Breakfast	
AM Snack	
Lunch	
PM Snack	
Dinner	
Drinks	

ACTIVITIES & OTHER COMMENTS

Appointments: _____

Health Concerns: _____

Plans For Tommorow: _____

Pain Level: _____ Happiness Level: _____ Alertness Level: _____

Supplies Needed Soon: _____

Medication Taken: _____

NOTES

Caregiving Notes For: _____ **Date:** _____ / _____ / _____

Toileting	Time								
	U								
	BM								

Times up During The Night				

Breakfast	
AM Snack	
Lunch	
PM Snack	
Dinner	
Drinks	

ACTIVITIES & OTHER COMMENTS

Appointments: _____

Health Concerns: _____

Plans For Tommorow: _____

Pain Level: _____ Happiness Level: _____ Alertness Level: _____

Supplies Needed Soon: _____

Medication Taken: _____

NOTES

Caregiving Notes For: _____   **Date:** _____ / _____ /

Toileting	Time						
	U						
	BM						

Times up During The Night				

Breakfast	
AM Snack	
Lunch	
PM Snack	
Dinner	
Drinks	

ACTIVITIES & OTHER COMMENTS

Appointments: _____

Health Concerns: _____

Plans For Tommorow: _____

Pain Level: _____ Happiness Level: _____ Alertness Level: _____

Supplies Needed Soon: _____

Medication Taken: _____

NOTES

Caregiving Notes For: _____ Date: ____/____/____

Toileting	Time							
	U							
	BM							

Times up During The Night

Breakfast	
AM Snack	
Lunch	
PM Snack	
Dinner	
Drinks	

ACTIVITIES & OTHER COMMENTS

Appointments: _____

Health Concerns: _____

Plans For Tommorow: _____

Pain Level: _____ Happiness Level: _____ Alertness Level: _____

Supplies Needed Soon: _____

Medication Taken: _____

NOTES

Caregiving Notes For: _____ **Date:** ____ / ____ / ____

Toileting	Time							
	U							
	BM							

Times up During The Night				

Breakfast	
AM Snack	
Lunch	
PM Snack	
Dinner	
Drinks	

ACTIVITIES & OTHER COMMENTS

Appointments: _____

Health Concerns: _____

Plans For Tommorow: _____

Pain Level: _____ Happiness Level: _____ Alertness Level: _____

Supplies Needed Soon: _____

Medication Taken: _____

NOTES

Caregiving Notes For: _____ Date: _____ / _____ / _____

Toileting	Time						
	U						
	BM						

Times up During The Night				

Breakfast	
AM Snack	
Lunch	
PM Snack	
Dinner	
Drinks	

ACTIVITIES & OTHER COMMENTS

Appointments: _____

Health Concerns: _____

Plans For Tommorow: _____

Pain Level: _____ Happiness Level: _____ Alertness Level: _____

Supplies Needed Soon: _____

Medication Taken: _____

NOTES

Caregiving Notes For: _____ Date: _____ / _____ / _____

Toileting	Time							
	U							
	BM							

Times up During The Night				

Breakfast	
AM Snack	
Lunch	
PM Snack	
Dinner	
Drinks	

ACTIVITIES & OTHER COMMENTS

Appointments: _____

Health Concerns: _____

Plans For Tommorow: _____

Pain Level: _____ Happiness Level: _____ Alertness Level: _____

Supplies Needed Soon: _____

Medication Taken: _____

NOTES

Caregiving Notes For: .... Date: ...... / ...... / ......

Toileting	Time						
	U						
	BM						

Times up During The Night				

Breakfast	
AM Snack	
Lunch	
PM Snack	
Dinner	
Drinks	

ACTIVITIES & OTHER COMMENTS

Appointments: ....

Health Concerns: ....

Plans For Tommorow: ....

Pain Level: .... Happiness Level: .... Alertness Level: ....

Supplies Needed Soon: ....

Medication Taken: ....

NOTES

Caregiving Notes For: _____ Date: _____ / _____ / _____

Toileting	Time							
	U							
	BM							

Times up During The Night | | | | |

Breakfast	
AM Snack	
Lunch	
PM Snack	
Dinner	
Drinks	

ACTIVITIES & OTHER COMMENTS

Appointments: _____

Health Concerns: _____

Plans For Tommorow: _____

Pain Level: _____ Happiness Level: _____ Alertness Level: _____

Supplies Needed Soon: _____

Medication Taken: _____

NOTES

Caregiving Notes For: _____ **Date:** ____ / ____ / ____

Toileting								
	Time							
	U							
	BM							

Times up During The Night				

Breakfast	
AM Snack	
Lunch	
PM Snack	
Dinner	
Drinks	

ACTIVITIES & OTHER COMMENTS

Appointments: _____

Health Concerns: _____

Plans For Tommorow: _____

Pain Level: _____ Happiness Level: _____ Alertness Level: _____

Supplies Needed Soon: _____

Medication Taken: _____

NOTES

Caregiving Notes For: _____ **Date:** ____ / ____ / ____

Toileting								
	Time							
	U							
	BM							

Times up During The Night				

Breakfast	
AM Snack	
Lunch	
PM Snack	
Dinner	
Drinks	

ACTIVITIES & OTHER COMMENTS

Appointments: _____

Health Concerns: _____

Plans For Tommorow: _____

Pain Level: _____ Happiness Level: _____ Alertness Level: _____

Supplies Needed Soon: _____

Medication Taken: _____

NOTES

Caregiving Notes For: .... **Date:** _____ / _____ / _____

Toileting	Time								
	U								
	BM								

Times up During The Night				

Breakfast	
AM Snack	
Lunch	
PM Snack	
Dinner	
Drinks	

ACTIVITIES & OTHER COMMENTS

Appointments: ....

Health Concerns: ....

Plans For Tommorow: ....

Pain Level: .... Happiness Level: .... Alertness Level: ....

Supplies Needed Soon: ....

Medication Taken: ....

NOTES

Caregiving Notes For: .... **Date:** _____ / _____ / _____

Toileting	Time							
	U							
	BM							

Times up During The Night				

Breakfast	
AM Snack	
Lunch	
PM Snack	
Dinner	
Drinks	

ACTIVITIES & OTHER COMMENTS

Appointments: ....

Health Concerns: ....

Plans For Tommorow: ....

Pain Level: .... Happiness Level: .... Alertness Level: ....

Supplies Needed Soon: ....

Medication Taken: ....

NOTES

Caregiving Notes For: .... **Date:** .... / .... / ....

Toileting	Time							
	U							
	BM							

Times up During The Night | | | |

Breakfast	
AM Snack	
Lunch	
PM Snack	
Dinner	
Drinks	

ACTIVITIES & OTHER COMMENTS

Appointments: ....

Health Concerns: ....

Plans For Tommorow: ....

Pain Level: .... Happiness Level: .... Alertness Level: ....

Supplies Needed Soon: ....

Medication Taken: ....

NOTES

Caregiving Notes For: _____ **Date:** ____ / ____ / ____

Toileting	Time							
	U							
	BM							

Times up During The Night				

Breakfast	
AM Snack	
Lunch	
PM Snack	
Dinner	
Drinks	

ACTIVITIES & OTHER COMMENTS

Appointments: _____

Health Concerns: _____

Plans For Tommorow: _____

Pain Level: _____ Happiness Level: _____ Alertness Level: _____

Supplies Needed Soon: _____

Medication Taken: _____

NOTES

Caregiving Notes For: _____ **Date:** ____ / ____ / ____

Toileting									
	Time								
	U								
	BM								

Times up During The Night				

Breakfast	
AM Snack	
Lunch	
PM Snack	
Dinner	
Drinks	

ACTIVITIES & OTHER COMMENTS

Appointments: _____

Health Concerns: _____

Plans For Tommorow: _____

Pain Level: _____ Happiness Level: _____ Alertness Level: _____

Supplies Needed Soon: _____

Medication Taken: _____

NOTES

Caregiving Notes For: _____   **Date:** _____ / _____ / _____

Toileting	Time							
	U							
	BM							

Times up During The Night				

Breakfast	
AM Snack	
Lunch	
PM Snack	
Dinner	
Drinks	

ACTIVITIES & OTHER COMMENTS

_____
_____
_____
_____
_____

Appointments: _____

Health Concerns: _____

Plans For Tommorow: _____

Pain Level: _____ Happiness Level: _____ Alertness Level: _____

Supplies Needed Soon: _____

Medication Taken: _____

NOTES

_____
_____
_____
_____

Caregiving Notes For: _____ Date: ____ / ____ / ____

Toileting									
	Time								
	U								
	BM								

Times up During The Night				

Breakfast	
AM Snack	
Lunch	
PM Snack	
Dinner	
Drinks	

ACTIVITIES & OTHER COMMENTS

Appointments: _____

Health Concerns: _____

Plans For Tommorow: _____

Pain Level: _____ Happiness Level: _____ Alertness Level: _____

Supplies Needed Soon: _____

Medication Taken: _____

NOTES

Caregiving Notes For: _____ Date: _____ / _____ / _____

Toileting	Time							
	U							
	BM							

Times up During The Night				

Breakfast	
AM Snack	
Lunch	
PM Snack	
Dinner	
Drinks	

ACTIVITIES & OTHER COMMENTS

Appointments: _____

Health Concerns: _____

Plans For Tommorow: _____

Pain Level: _____ Happiness Level: _____ Alertness Level: _____

Supplies Needed Soon: _____

Medication Taken: _____

NOTES

Caregiving Notes For: ....   Date: .... / .... / ....

Toileting	Time						
	U						
	BM						

Times up During The Night				

Breakfast	
AM Snack	
Lunch	
PM Snack	
Dinner	
Drinks	

ACTIVITIES & OTHER COMMENTS

Appointments: ....

Health Concerns: ....

Plans For Tommorow: ....

Pain Level: .... Happiness Level: .... Alertness Level: ....

Supplies Needed Soon: ....

Medication Taken: ....

NOTES

Caregiving Notes For: _____   **Date:** ____ / ____ / ____

Toileting	Time							
	U							
	BM							

Times up During The Night				

Breakfast	
AM Snack	
Lunch	
PM Snack	
Dinner	
Drinks	

ACTIVITIES & OTHER COMMENTS

Appointments: _____

Health Concerns: _____

Plans For Tommorow: _____

Pain Level: _____ Happiness Level: _____ Alertness Level: _____

Supplies Needed Soon: _____

Medication Taken: _____

NOTES

Caregiving Notes For: _____ **Date:** _____ / _____ / _____

Toileting							
	Time						
	U						
	BM						

Times up During The Night				

Breakfast	
AM Snack	
Lunch	
PM Snack	
Dinner	
Drinks	

ACTIVITIES & OTHER COMMENTS

Appointments: _____

Health Concerns: _____

Plans For Tommorow: _____

Pain Level: _____ Happiness Level: _____ Alertness Level: _____

Supplies Needed Soon: _____

Medication Taken: _____

NOTES

Caregiving Notes For: _____ **Date:** ____ / ____ / ____

Toileting	Time						
	U						
	BM						

Times up During The Night				

Breakfast	
AM Snack	
Lunch	
PM Snack	
Dinner	
Drinks	

ACTIVITIES & OTHER COMMENTS

Appointments: _____

Health Concerns: _____

Plans For Tommorow: _____

Pain Level: _____ Happiness Level: _____ Alertness Level: _____

Supplies Needed Soon: _____

Medication Taken: _____

NOTES

Caregiving Notes For: .... **Date:** .... / .... / ....

Toileting	Time							
	U							
	BM							

Times up During The Night				

Breakfast	
AM Snack	
Lunch	
PM Snack	
Dinner	
Drinks	

ACTIVITIES & OTHER COMMENTS

Appointments: ....

Health Concerns: ....

Plans For Tommorow: ....

Pain Level: .... Happiness Level: .... Alertness Level: ....

Supplies Needed Soon: ....

Medication Taken: ....

NOTES

Caregiving Notes For: .... Date: ...... / ...... / ......

Toileting	Time						
	U						
	BM						

Times up During The Night				

Breakfast	
AM Snack	
Lunch	
PM Snack	
Dinner	
Drinks	

ACTIVITIES & OTHER COMMENTS

Appointments: ....

Health Concerns: ....

Plans For Tommorow: ....

Pain Level: .... Happiness Level: .... Alertness Level: ....

Supplies Needed Soon: ....

Medication Taken: ....

NOTES

Caregiving Notes For: _____ **Date:** _____ / _____ / _____

Toileting	Time							
	U							
	BM							

Times up During The Night			

Breakfast	
AM Snack	
Lunch	
PM Snack	
Dinner	
Drinks	

ACTIVITIES & OTHER COMMENTS

Appointments: _____

Health Concerns: _____

Plans For Tommorow: _____

Pain Level: _____ Happiness Level: _____ Alertness Level: _____

Supplies Needed Soon: _____

Medication Taken: _____

NOTES

Caregiving Notes For: .... **Date:** .... / .... / ....

Toileting								
	Time							
	U							
	BM							

Times up During The Night				

Breakfast	
AM Snack	
Lunch	
PM Snack	
Dinner	
Drinks	

ACTIVITIES & OTHER COMMENTS

Appointments: ....

Health Concerns: ....

Plans For Tommorow: ....

Pain Level: .... Happiness Level: .... Alertness Level: ....

Supplies Needed Soon: ....

Medication Taken: ....

NOTES

Caregiving Notes For: _____ **Date:** ___/___/___

<table>
<tr><td rowspan="3">Toileting</td><td>Time</td><td></td><td></td><td></td><td></td><td></td><td></td></tr>
<tr><td>U</td><td></td><td></td><td></td><td></td><td></td><td></td></tr>
<tr><td>BM</td><td></td><td></td><td></td><td></td><td></td><td></td></tr>
</table>

Times up During The Night				

Breakfast	
AM Snack	
Lunch	
PM Snack	
Dinner	
Drinks	

ACTIVITIES & OTHER COMMENTS

Appointments: _____

Health Concerns: _____

Plans For Tommorow: _____

Pain Level: _____ Happiness Level: _____ Alertness Level: _____

Supplies Needed Soon: _____

Medication Taken: _____

NOTES

Caregiving Notes For: _____   **Date:** _____ / _____ / _____

Toileting	Time								
	U								
	BM								

Times up During The Night				

Breakfast	
AM Snack	
Lunch	
PM Snack	
Dinner	
Drinks	

ACTIVITIES & OTHER COMMENTS

Appointments: _____

Health Concerns: _____

Plans For Tommorow: _____

Pain Level: _____ Happiness Level: _____ Alertness Level: _____

Supplies Needed Soon: _____

Medication Taken: _____

NOTES

Caregiving Notes For: _____   **Date:** ____ / ____ / ____

Toileting	Time						
	U						
	BM						

Times up During The Night				

Breakfast	
AM Snack	
Lunch	
PM Snack	
Dinner	
Drinks	

ACTIVITIES & OTHER COMMENTS

Appointments: _____

Health Concerns: _____

Plans For Tommorow: _____

Pain Level: _____   Happiness Level: _____   Alertness Level: _____

Supplies Needed Soon: _____

Medication Taken: _____

NOTES

Dear Caregiver

Producing this book was a one-man operation,
and it took a lot of hard work to bring this quality to you.
If you like this book, please spend a moment
to add a review on amazon.com, this will help
others to find the book.

I am **forever** grateful for your support.

Thank You

Made in the USA
Middletown, DE
16 March 2024

51607991R00077